PREPARIN

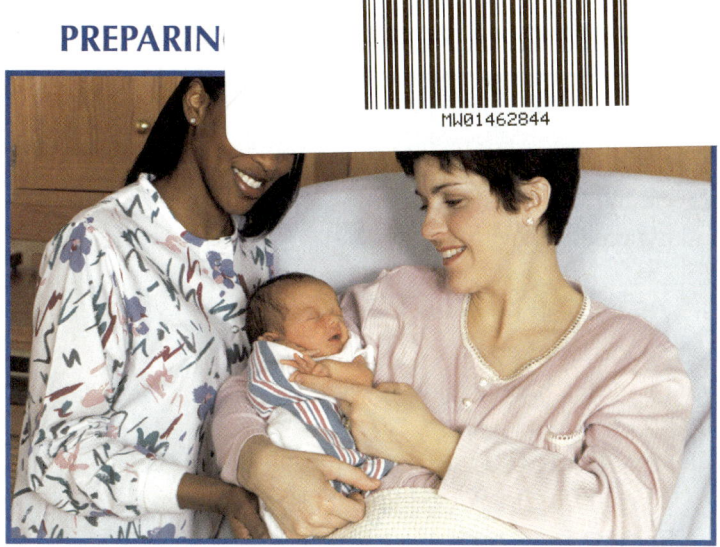

This booklet was written in collaboration with:

Linda Mayberry, RN, PhD, FAAN, Associate Professor
New York University, NY

Susan Gennaro, DSN, FAAN, Professor
University of Pennsylvania, Philadelphia, PA

We gratefully acknowledge the perinatal nurses from the following hospitals who participated in the Upright Positioning in Labor Education Project, which is the basis for this booklet.

Brigham & Women's Hospital, Boston, MA
Mercy Fitzgerald Hospital, Darby, PA
Miami Valley Hospital, Dayton, OH
New York University Hospital, New York, NY
St. Joseph Health Center, London, Ontario

Additional contributions by Polly Perez, RN, BSN

The information contained in this book is general. It is not intended to replace the advice and recommendations of your health care provider. Consult your health care provider if you have a question or concern.

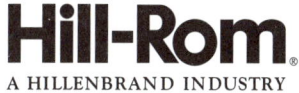

© 2002 Care Publications, Inc.

1

TABLE OF CONTENTS

PREGNANCY CARE

Anatomy of pregnancy	6
Healthy eating during pregnancy	7
Food pyramid, Eating tips, Eating out	
Weight gain	8
Healthy exercise and fitness during pregnancy	9
The importance of exercise	
Exercise during pregnancy	
ACOG fitness exercises	10
Upper Body Bend, Diagonal Curl, Forward Bend, Trunk Twist, Backward Stretch, Leg Lift Crawl, Rocking Back Arch, Back Press	
Labor ball suggestions	
First trimester	14
Sitting, Seated slow bounce, Side-to-side sitting	
Second trimester	15
Circular sitting, Lying rest, Lying roll	
Third trimester	17
Leg squeeze	
Decisions before you deliver	
To do checklist	18
Planning for labor and delivery visitors	19
Shopping lists for you and baby	20
What to bring to the hospital	21

LABOR AND BIRTH

Signs that labor is near	24
About labor	25
True vs. false labor	
Knowing when you're in labor	26
Coming to the hospital	27
Admission	
Your care team	

Comfort measures for labor and birth	28
Hydrotherapy	28
Aromatherapy	28
Sterile water injections	28
Positions for Labor	29
Double hip squeeze, Knee pressure, Back counter pressure, Over head of bed, Lunge, Epidural anesthesia	
Using the birth ball with the bed	31
Sitting on ball, Lying on ball, Leaning on ball	
Using a peanut ball	32
Positions for Birth	33
Saddle, Throne	
Using a labor bar	34
Tug of war, Squatting	
Dangle squat, Side-lying	35
Labor and the birth of your baby	36
Stages of labor: Changes, What to expect, What your support person can do	
First stage: Early phase, Active phase, Transition phase	37
Second stage	40
Third stage	40
Assisted delivery	41
Inducing (Starting) labor, Pitocin (Oxytocin), Rupture of membrane, Vacuum and forceps	
Cesarean birth	42
When a Cesarean is needed, After your Cesarean Vaginal birth after cesarean (VBAC)	
Care at birth for vaginal, VBAC, C-section	43
Mother's recovery care	43
Baby's medical care at birth	44
While in the hospital	45
Infant security, Birth certificate and Social Security number	45

3

Mom's care at home 46
    Emotions and depression 47
    Warning signs 48
Nutrition after the birth 49
Activity level and exercise after delivery 49
    ACOG fitness exercises 50
        Leg slides, Head lifts, Shoulder lifts,
        Curl-ups, Kneeling pelvic tilt
    Kegel exercises 53
    Birth ball exercises postpartum 54
        Pelvic lift exercise, lunge

APPENDICES

Food Pyramid for Women and Families 58
    Pregnant, Breastfeeding, Postpartum, Teen Mothers
Glossary 60

INDEX 63

YOUR PREGNANCY HEALTH

YOUR PREGNANCY HEALTH

The female body is designed by nature to accommodate the growth and development of new life. Hormone levels rise or fall. Energy levels come and go. Organs shift to make room for the fetus as it grows and develops.

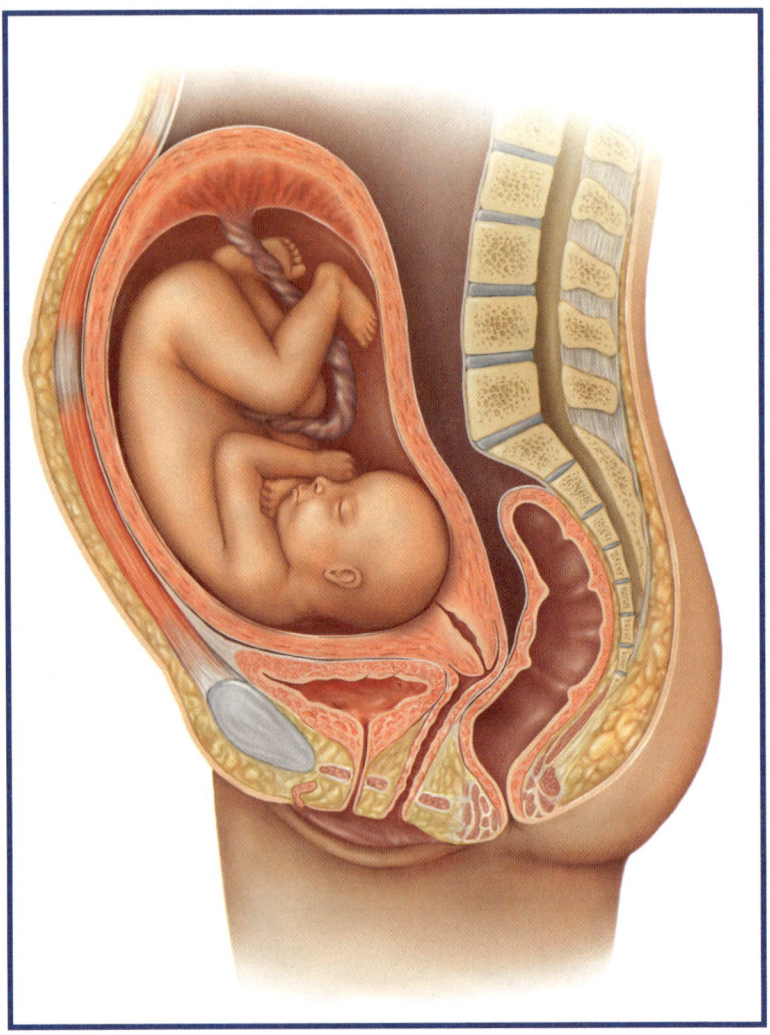

HEALTHY EATING

One of the best things a mother can do during pregnancy for herself and her baby is to eat well. It's not hard to do, and it doesn't cost a lot of money. The right food will help give your baby a terrific start.

FOOD PYRAMID

The food pyramid in Appendix A, page 58, shows the number of servings recommended for pregnant women. Talk with your health care provider to see if you may have special dietary needs.

SOME EATING TIPS

Eating good food will help you and your baby stay healthy. Some tips:

- Drink lots of liquids—water, milk, juices. Try to have 6 to 8 glasses daily.
- Cut down on fried foods, candy bars, soft drinks, doughnuts, pastries, and other foods high in sugar or fat.
- Try to snack on healthy foods like fruits, vegetables, cereal, yogurt, or cheese.

EATING OUT

When you go to a restaurant, you can still eat well. Eating right does not cost more, and it tastes great.

- Order plain burgers and cheeseburgers, topped with ketchup or mustard only. Avoid extra sauces and toppings like mayonnaise, tartar sauce, and bacon.
- Choose baked, broiled, or grilled foods, instead of fried foods. Avoid undercooked meat.
- Skip the French fries. Instead, get a plain baked potato.
- Salads that have meat or seafood and cheese are great meals. Side salads help you get the vegetables you and your baby need.
- Ask for low-calorie salad dressings.
- Stay away from fatty meats—bacon, sausage, hot dogs, pepperoni, and salami.
- Stick with meatless pizzas that have cheese and vegetable toppings only.
- Turkey, chicken, and roast beef submarines, loaded with vegetables, are good.
- Choose milk or fruit juice rather than soda.

WEIGHT GAIN

The weight you gain is distributed around your body this way:

Baby	7 to 8 pounds
Changes in mother's body:	
Breast increase	1 to 2 pounds
Blood increase	4 to 5 pounds
Fat	5 to 7 pounds
Body fluid	1 to 2 pounds
Uterus increase	2 to 5 pounds
Placenta	2 to 3 pounds
Amniotic fluid	2 to 3 pounds
Total	25 to 35 pounds

ABOUT YOUR WEIGHT

Eating the right foods will help you make sure you do not gain too little weight or too much.

Gaining weight sometimes makes pregnant women feel unhappy or uncomfortable. But a steady weight gain is important to the health of your baby. While the average newborn weighs about 7 pounds, you must gain much more than that to support your baby's development. Besides, many women lose the extra weight they have gained within six weeks to six months after their baby is born.

Remember: you're not getting fat. You're helping your unborn child have a healthy start in life.

- Expect to gain 3 or 4 pounds during the first three months of your pregnancy.
- From your fourth month on, you will gain about a pound a week.
- The average weight gain for the entire pregnancy is 25 to 35 pounds. Your health care provider may advise you to gain more or less.
- Do not try to lose weight while you're pregnant, no matter how heavy you are. This could hurt your baby. Talk with your provider about an appropriate meal plan.

HEALTHY EXERCISE AND FITNESS DURING PREGNANCY

THE IMPORTANCE OF EXERCISE

Regular exercise may not only make you look better during pregnancy—it may make you feel better too. It can lessen fatigue, relieve stress, improve your posture, and help with backaches.

Always check with your health care provider about exercises you wish to do.

You'll do yourself a favor if you get a moderate amount of regular exercise on most, if not all, days of the week. Walking and swimming are excellent types of exercise for pregnant women. Almost every kind of exercise is safe, as long as you are careful and don't try to do too much.

- Use your common sense and stay away from sports that could cause you to fall and hurt yourself and your baby.

- Drink lots of water before, during, and after your exercise. It's important that you take in enough fluids.

- Avoid temperature extremes, especially heat.

- Now is not the time to lose weight. You should exercise only to keep yourself fit—you can lose weight after the baby is born.

- Avoid jumping and jarring your body. Remember that your joints are looser now, so be extra careful not to strain yourself. Plus, your center of gravity shifts as you become more and more pregnant, making you more likely to fall.

- If you have any of these warning signals, stop exercising and call your care provider:

  - Pain
  - Vaginal bleeding
  - Shortness of breath
  - Irregular or rapid heart beat
  - Difficulty in walking
  - Pain in your back or pubic area
  - Dizziness or feeling faint

Remember to get up from the floor slowly to prevent dizziness.

PREGNANCY FITNESS EXERCISES SUGGESTED BY ACOG

These 8 fitness exercises are suggested by the American College of Obstetricians and Gynecologists for pregnant women. However, you should always consult your care provider before you begin any personal fitness or exercise program.

American College of Obstetricians and Gynecologists: Planning for Pregnancy, Birth and Beyond, Second Edition © 1995 and Third Edition © 2000. Washington, DC, ACOG. Used with permission.

UPPER BODY BEND

To strengthen the muscles of your back and torso.

- Stand with your legs apart, knees bent slightly, with your hands on your hips.
- Bend forward slowly, keeping your upper back straight. You should feel a slight pull along your upper thigh.
- Repeat 10 times.

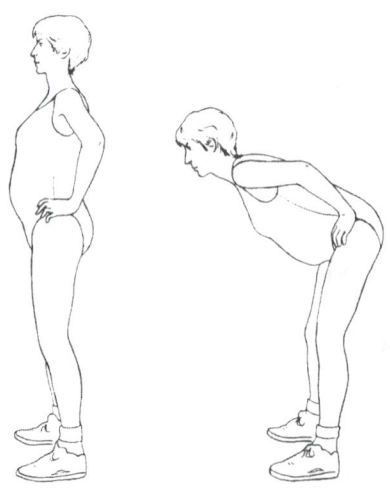

DIAGONAL CURL

To strengthen the muscles of your back, hips, and abdomen. If you have not already been exercising regularly, skip this exercise.

- Sit on the floor with your knees bent, feet on the floor, and hands clasped in front of you.
- Twist your upper torso to the left until your hands touch the floor.
- Do the same movement to the right.
- Repeat on both sides 5 times.

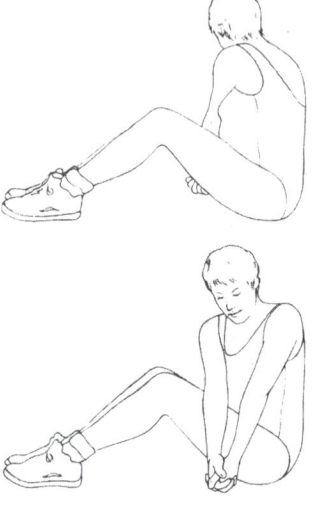

FORWARD BEND

To stretch and strengthen the muscles of your back.

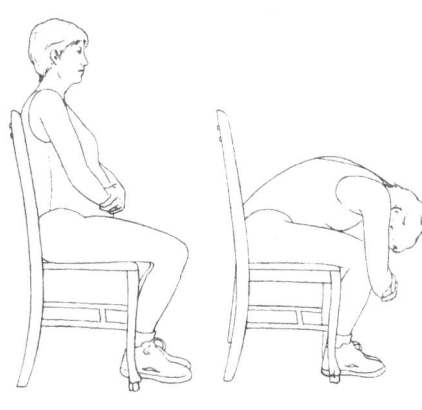

- Sit in a chair in a comfortable position. Keep your arms relaxed.
- Bend forward slowly, with your arms in front and hanging down.
- If you feel any discomfort or pressure on your abdomen, do not push any further.
- Hold this position for a count of 5, then sit up slowly without arching your back.
- Repeat 5 times.

TRUNK TWIST

To stretch the muscles of your back, spine, and upper torso.

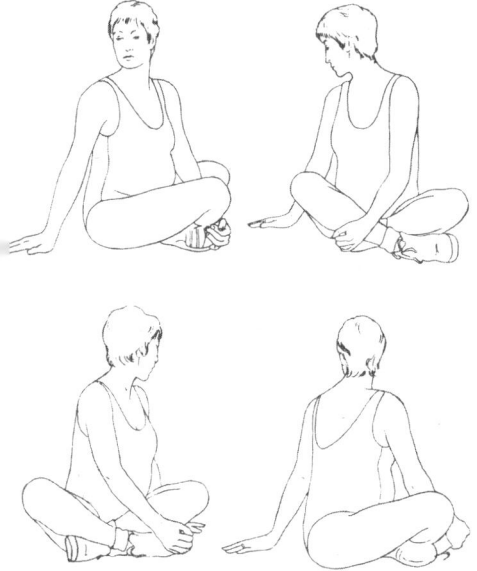

- Sit on the floor with your legs crossed, with your left hand holding your left foot and your right hand on the floor at your side for support.
- Slowly twist your upper torso to the right.
- Do the same movement to the left, after switching your hands (right hand holding right foot and left hand supporting you).
- Repeat on both sides 5 to 10 times.

BACKWARD STRETCH

To stretch and strengthen the muscles of your back, pelvis, and thighs.

- Kneel on hands and knees, with your knees 8 to 10 inches apart and your arms straight (hands under your shoulders).

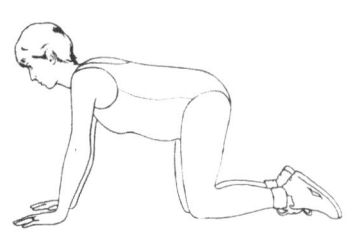

- Curl backward slowly, tucking your head toward your knees and keeping your arms extended.

- Hold this position for a count of 5, then come back up to all fours slowly.

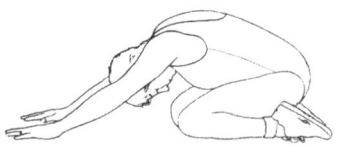

- Repeat 5 times.

LEG LIFT CRAWL

To strengthen the muscles of your back and abdomen.

- Kneel on hands and knees, with your weight distributed evenly and your arms straight (hands under your shoulders).

- Lift your left knee and bring it toward your elbow.

- Straighten your leg without locking your knee.

- Extend your leg up and back.

- Do this exercise to a count of 5. Move slowly; don't fling your leg back or arch your back.

- Repeat on both sides 5 to 10 times.

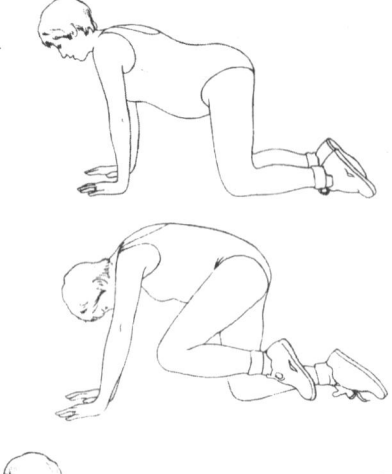

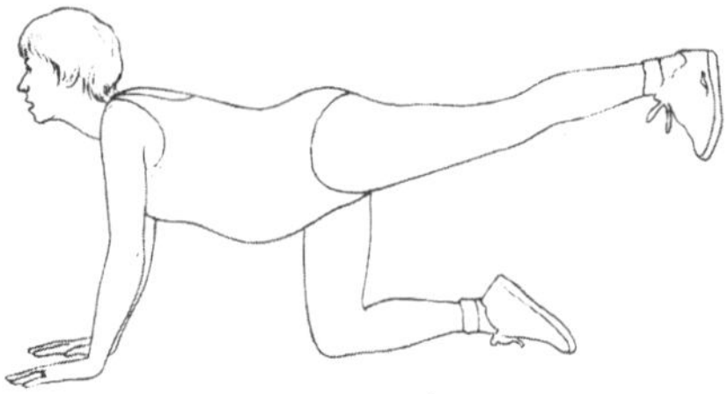

ROCKING BACK ARCH

To stretch and strengthen the muscles of your back, hips, and abdomen.

- Kneel on hands and knees, with your weight distributed evenly and your back straight.
- Rock back and forth to a count of 5.
- Return to the original position and curl your back upward as much as you can.
- Repeat 5 to 10 times.

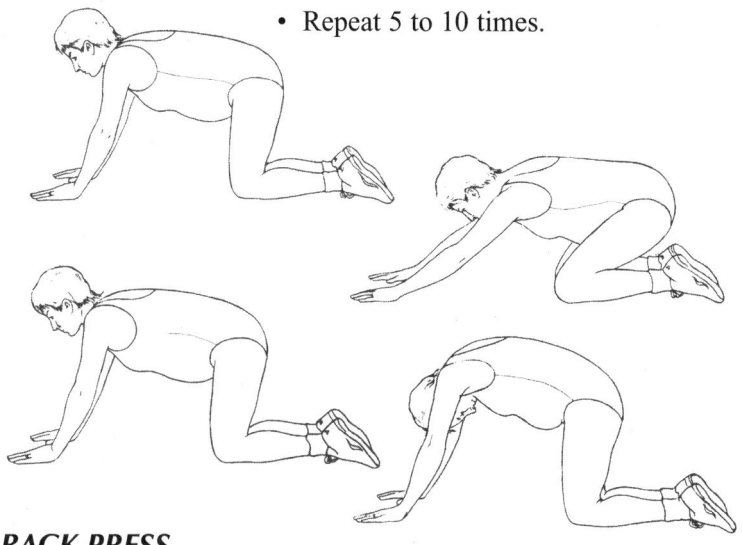

BACK PRESS

To strengthen the muscles of your back, torso, and upper body and promote good posture.

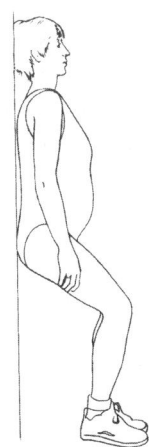

- Stand with your feet 10 to 12 inches away from a wall and your back against it.
- Press the lower part of your back against the wall.
- Hold this position for a count of 10, then release.
- Repeat 10 times.

PREGNANCY FITNESS EXERCISES USING A LABOR BALL

Some childbirth specialists recommend that pregnant women can exercise with a large ball. You should attend classes or talk with a specially trained health care professional to learn how to use the ball for prenatal and childbirth exercises. These specialists can help you get the right size ball, which depends on your height. They can teach you how to use the ball safely. You can brace yourself with a nearby wall or piece of furniture until you are comfortable using the ball alone. Another person can also stand behind you.

Ball exercises can relieve back pain and tone the abdominal muscles used in childbirth. The ball can also strengthen the pelvic floor, which is stressed during pregnancy and delivery.

FIRST TRIMESTER

The body's center of gravity changes during pregnancy. These exercises can promote good posture, prevent low back pain, and stimulate blood flow.

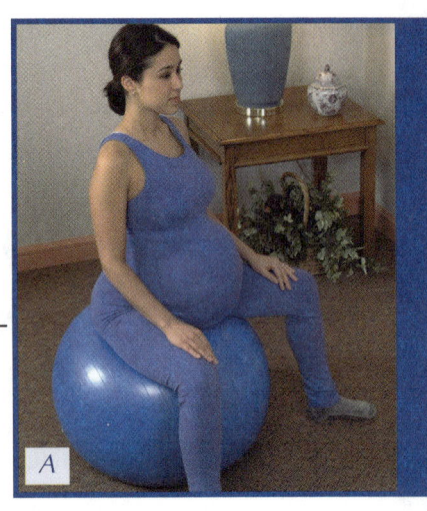

Sitting. Practice sitting on the ball with upper body erect, arms and shoulders relaxed, hands resting on thighs. Legs are bent and slightly apart, feet firmly on the floor. *Fig. A*

Seated slow bounce. Sit on the ball with feet firmly on the floor and legs bent, slightly apart. Keep the upper body naturally erect, the arms and shoulders relaxed. Slightly tilt the pelvis backward. Begin a slow, continuous bouncing movement, keeping the pelvis in contact with the ball, for about 1 minute. *Fig. A*

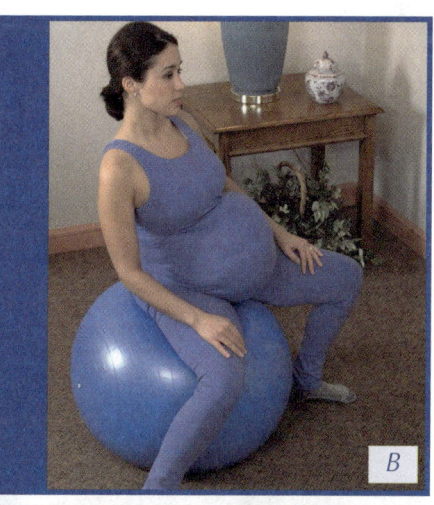

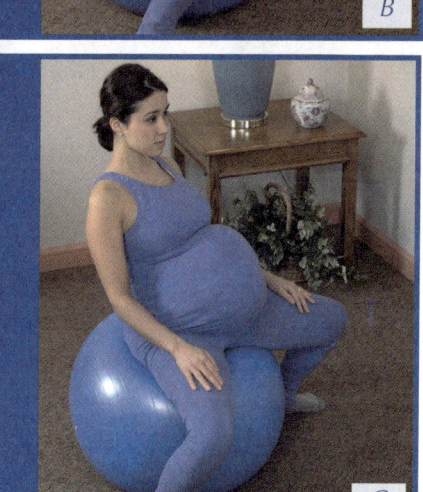

Side-to-side movements. Sit on the ball, feet apart, hands on thighs. Breathe naturally. Gently move hips slightly from one side to the other, matching the movement to your breathing. *Fig. B*

SECOND TRIMESTER

These exercises may help strengthen the abdominal muscles and improve mobility of the pelvis.

Circular sitting. Sit on the ball, feet apart, hands on thighs. Tilt pelvis slightly backward and push with leg to make slow, continuous circular movements of the pelvis. Do the same movement in the opposite direction. Repeat for 15 to 20 seconds. *Fig. A and C*

SECOND TRIMESTER
(continued)

Lying rest. Lie on your back on the floor, arms extended, palms down. Place ball under calves of legs with legs slightly bent. *Fig. A*

Note: Do not lie on your back for long periods of time. If you feel dizzy or sick, roll to the side and discontinue. The weight of the baby may be blocking blood flow.

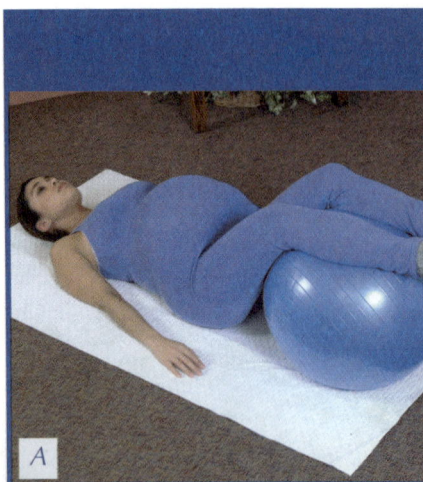

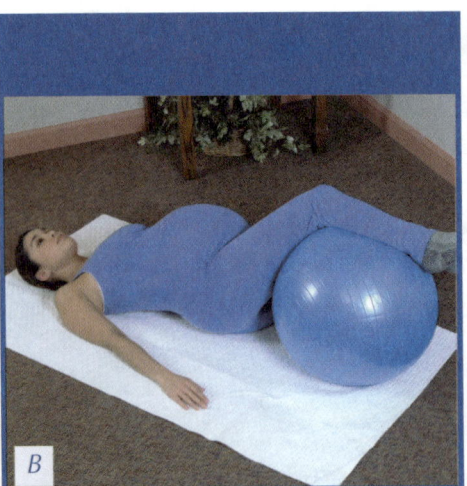

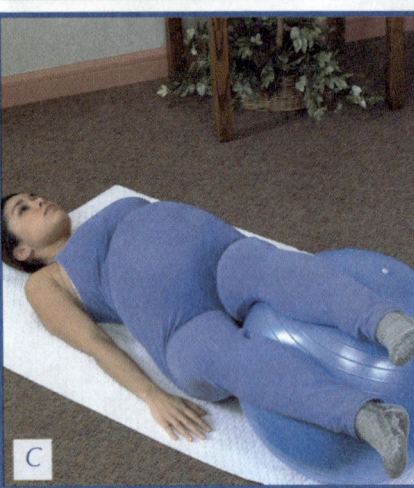

Lying roll. Lie on the floor on your back, arms by your sides, palms down. Legs are bent and slightly apart, resting on the top of the ball. Turn feet slightly inward and rotate the ball from the central position to the right, return to center, then to the left. Breathe out when moving the ball to the left or right. Breathe in when returning to center. *Fig. B and C*

THIRD TRIMESTER

This exercise may increase awareness of tension and improve ability to relax the muscles in the pelvis, legs, and diaphragm.

Leg squeeze. Sit naturally erect on the floor with your arms behind you to provide stability. Legs are bent and slightly apart, feet resting on the floor. Place the ball between your knees. Take a deep breath while squeezing the ball with the legs for a few seconds. Then exhale deeply while relaxing the leg muscles.
Fig. D and E

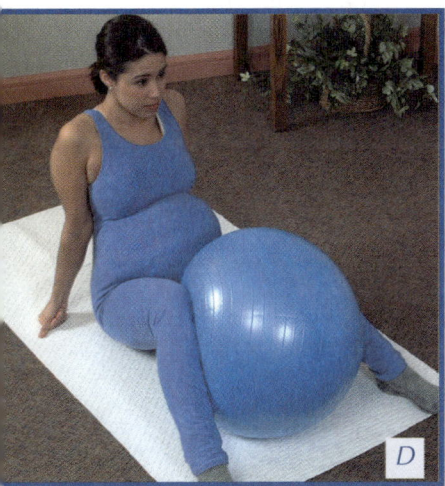
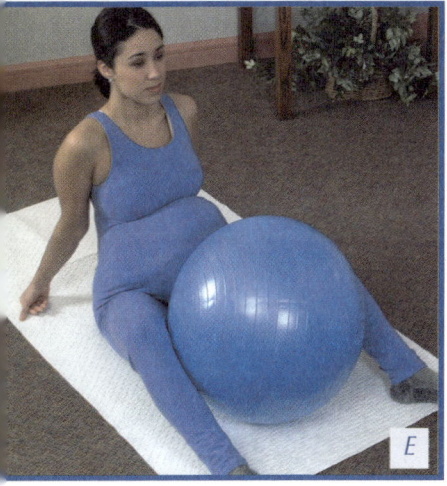

DECISIONS BEFORE YOU DELIVER

A little planning goes a long way. Plan for your stay before you go to the hospital. You'll need some supplies at home, too, to care for your new baby. The list below should help.

TO-DO CHECKLIST TO GET YOURSELF READY FOR DELIVERY

- ❑ Plan your hospital trip. Take into account the time of day, traffic, and weather. If a ride to the hospital is a problem, make arrangements long before you go into labor.
- ❑ Be sure you understand what you should do when labor begins.
    - Ask your care provider when to call.
    - Ask how you reach your care provider after office hours.
- ❑ Have your bag packed and ready to go.
- ❑ Arrange child care for siblings while you are in the hospital.
- ❑ Do you have pets that will need attention?
- ❑ Know your plans about family planning and spacing your children following delivery.
- ❑ Decide on the baby's name for the birth certificate and for the Social Security number.
- ❑ Get your baby's car seat for the ride home from the hospital.
- ❑ Prepare a few meals ahead that freeze well to use when you come home from the hospital.
- ❑ Choose your baby's care provider now so that he or she can examine the baby during the hospital stay.
- ❑ Decide, if your newborn is male, if you want him circumcised. Discuss risks and benefits with your health care provider.
- ❑ Even if you plan to deliver naturally, explore pain therapy options with your care provider. Discuss risks and benefits so you can be prepared to make an informed decision.

PLANNING FOR LABOR AND DELIVERY VISITORS

We want you to know our visitor guidelines before you come to deliver your baby. They are for your safety, comfort, and care. Please review them with your family and support person(s) before delivery.

Remember, too, that while you are in labor and after the baby is born, you will be very busy. So will your care team, who will make sure you and your baby get all the medical attention you need. You may not have the time or energy for many visitors. You might ask some of them to wait until you go home to visit.

Prepare your children in advance for their visit with you after the baby arrives. Register them for a sibling preparation class before the birth. Children can not stay overnight with you while you are in the hospital.

PLANNING NOTES
(Visiting hours, phone numbers to remember, etc.)

SHOPPING LISTS FOR YOU AND BABY

Here are suggestions of what you may need to care for your new baby. Remember, babies grow so quickly that they only wear their clothes for a short time.

Linens and Things

- ❏ Crib that meets all safety regulations, including unleaded paint, slats no more than 2-3/8" apart, no corner posts
- ❏ Snug-fitting mattress and bumper pads (rolled-up blankets or towels will work)
- ❏ 3-4 fitted crib sheets, a blanket or quilt
- ❏ 3-4 waterproof pads
- ❏ 2-3 receiving blankets

Diaper Supplies

- ❏ Diapers (cloth or disposable)
- ❏ Waterproof pants if needed
- ❏ Diaper pail if using cloth diapers
- ❏ Diaper bag for supplies when you leave the house

Baby Clothes

- ❏ 4-6 undershirts or onesies (not necessary in warm weather)
- ❏ 4-6 gowns/sleepers
- ❏ 1-2 blanket sleepers (for cold weather)
- ❏ 4-6 outfits appropriate for the season
- ❏ Bunting/hat with warm blankets for cold weather
- ❏ 3 pair socks or booties
- ❏ 3 bibs
- ❏ 2 caps or bonnets

Formula-Feeding Supplies
(if you are not planning to breastfeed)

- ❏ 6-8 bottles
- ❏ 6-8 nipples
- ❏ Formula (2-week supply)

Medical Supplies and Bath Items

- ❏ Digital thermometer
- ❏ Mild soap
- ❏ Petroleum jelly
- ❏ Baby shampoo
- ❏ Rubbing alcohol
- ❏ Unscented baby products
- ❏ Cotton balls

For Mom

- ❏ Sanitary napkins
- ❏ Bra pads without plastic lining or homemade cotton pads if breastfeeding
- ❏ 2 nursing bras (optional)
- ❏ Mild pain reliever (Tylenol®, ibuprofen)
- ❏ Witch hazel pads (Tucks®)

Transportation

Car safety seat that meets federal safety standards. Take it to the hospital for baby's first ride home.

WHAT TO BRING TO THE HOSPITAL

Several weeks before your due date, pack a bag that will be ready to go to the hospital when you are. Here are some items you may want to include:

- ❏ Nightgown or pajamas that button down the front
- ❏ Robe and slippers
- ❏ Underwear—regular or nursing bras, panties
- ❏ Toiletries
- ❏ Loose-fitting clothes to wear home
- ❏ Clothes for baby to wear home, including shirt, pants, receiving blanket—look for fire-retardant clothing and bedding
- ❏ Health insurance card
- ❏ WIC forms
- ❏ Coins for vending machines
- ❏ List of numbers to call to announce the baby's arrival
- ❏ Camera loaded with film, fresh batteries, flash equipment

You may also want to pack a "goody bag" for labor. Here are some items you will want to include:

- ❏ Pillows
- ❏ Lip moisturizer such as Chapstick®
- ❏ Snack for coach
- ❏ Pad and pencil
- ❏ Battery-operated music source (radio, tape player)
- ❏ Childbirth class folder
- ❏ Focal point
- ❏ Tennis balls in sock
- ❏ Socks for mom

Please—do not bring jewelry or large sums of money to the hospital.

PLANNING NOTES

LABOR AND BIRTH

SIGNS THAT LABOR IS NEAR

Your due date is just a best guess of when your baby will be born. You may feel everything listed below, some of it, or none of it. Each labor is different.

- **Lightening.** The baby drops or settles into the pelvis during the last few weeks before labor begins. This may cause an increase in pelvic pressure and a frequent need to urinate.
- **Nesting.** You may feel an increase in energy and want to do more to prepare for the baby.
- **Bloody show.** You may notice a mucus-like discharge from the vagina with streaks of blood. It can happen after a vaginal exam or in the last days or weeks before birth.
- **Low backache.** May come and go, or pressure may be constant.
- **Bowel movement change.** Either diarrhea or constipation.
- **Effacement** (thinning of the cervix). This is noticed on exam by your care provider. Your cervix may also begin to open. Some thinning and opening of the cervix is common in the last weeks of pregnancy.
- **Bag of waters breaks** (membranes rupture). The water may come as a slow trickle of fluid from your vagina, or you may have a sudden gush. Consider putting a rubber mattress cover on your bed at home in case your membranes rupture while you are in bed. It may happen before or after contractions begin. If this happens, don't take a bath. Call your care provider.
- **Contractions.** During labor your uterus gets tight and then relaxes. Contractions feel like cramps. They help the baby move through the birth canal.

ABOUT LABOR

Labor is the work done by your uterus that results in the birth of your baby. No two deliveries are exactly alike, but the information below can give you an idea of what to expect.

Labor lasts an average of 12 to 20 hours for the first birth. If this is not your first birth, it may take less time.

KNOWING WHEN IT'S TRUE LABOR

As you get closer to your delivery date, you may feel minor contractions that can be painful. These are called *Braxton-Hicks* contractions, and they are perfectly normal. But they are not necessarily a sign that true labor has started.

If you have contractions that do not become closer together or stronger, and you have no other signs of labor, you are probably not in true labor yet.

True Labor	*False Labor*
• Contractions become longer, stronger, and grow closer together.	• Contractions usually stay the same.
• Contractions don't go away with rest and you cannot sleep through them.	• Labor may stop or become irregular with rest or a change in activity.
• The cervix continues to dilate and efface (open and get thinner).	• The cervix doesn't change.

KNOWING WHEN YOU'RE IN LABOR

Sometimes it's hard to tell if true labor has begun. The guidelines below should help you decide.

- For EVERYONE, call your care provider and come to the hospital if:
    - the bag of waters has broken or is leaking even a small amount
    - you see bleeding from your vagina. You do not need to come in if you have spotting of only pink or bloody mucus discharge.
    - If in doubt, call your care provider.

- If this is your FIRST baby, come to the hospital when:
    - labor pains (contractions) happen every 5 minutes

      AND
    - each one lasts 45 seconds or more

      AND
    - they have been like that for about 2 hours.

- If this is your SECOND (or third or more) baby, come to the hospital when:
    - labor pains are regular and happen every 10 minutes and are not relieved by rest.

IMPORTANT!

Before you leave for the hospital, call your health care provider to let him or her know you are coming.

Your care provider's phone number:

_____

Your hospital's phone number:

_____

COMING TO THE HOSPITAL

ADMISSION—WHAT TO EXPECT

If you are in true labor, you will be admitted for the delivery of your baby. When you enter the labor area, here's what happens:

- You will be asked to change into a hospital gown.
- You will be examined to determine how close you are to delivery.
- Soon after you are admitted, a nurse may place an intravenous (IV) needle attached to a tube into your arm or wrist. This IV will be used throughout labor, delivery, and recovery. Through it you will get fluids, medications (if needed), or blood (only if necessary).
- An electronic fetal monitoring device will be used to monitor your baby during your labor. This equipment records the unborn baby's heart rate and movements. It also shows the contractions of the uterus.
- You may not be able to eat or drink, but you may be allowed ice chips during labor.

YOUR CARE TEAM

Your care provider will check your progress periodically throughout your labor. A team of nurses who specialize in labor and delivery nursing will be at your side. They will monitor your heart rate, blood pressure, labor progress, and the baby's well-being.

This team specializes in the physical and emotional needs of families during labor and delivery. They will guide and support you and your family throughout this special time.

COMFORT MEASURES FOR LABOR AND BIRTH

There are a number of comfort measures and upright positions you can use that may help make labor and delivery easier and quicker. When you relax your muscles and lower your anxiety, you will also help labor progress. Here are some examples.

HYDROTHERAPY

Water—showers and baths—can help you relax, give relief from pain and enable you to keep moving, which in turn helps labor to progress. Water's warmth helps mother relax and support the pelvic floor muscles.

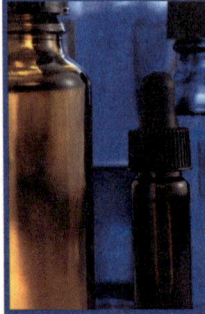

AROMATHERAPY

Some women may find that aromatherapy lowers their stress and anxiety. Essential oils of plants are used for massage, as a room spray, or drops on a pillow. Lavender can be relaxing. Peppermint may help stop nausea and vomiting.

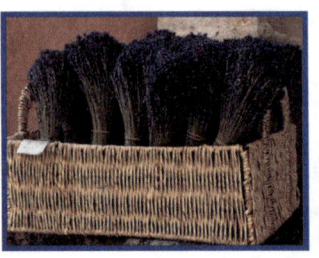

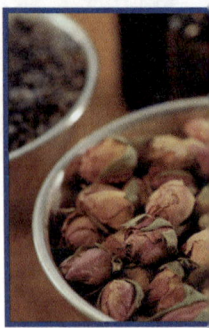

STERILE WATER INJECTIONS

A small amount of sterile water can be injected into the skin of the lower back for relief of pain. Its effects last 45 to 90 minutes. This can be a useful therapy for lower back pain.

POSITIONS FOR LABOR

Certain upright positions help your body work with (not against) the birthing process, making your baby's journey through the birth canal easier. Plus you may have less discomfort and feel in more control. *Fig. A*

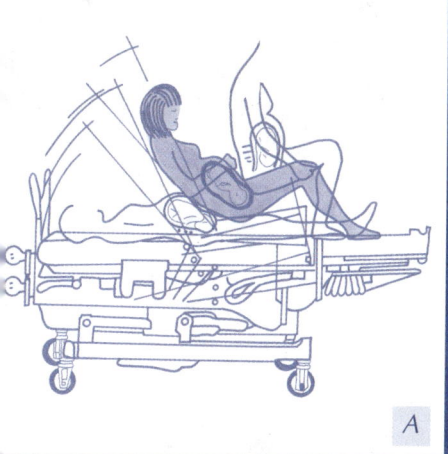

Work with your health care provider to identify positions you may use, particularly if you have an epidural when you may have less motor function.

DOUBLE HIP SQUEEZE

Shortens the ligament on the back and helps reduce back pain. Partner applies pressure on the hips with the heal of the hands, pressing the hips together, then upward. This may also be done using the birth ball. *Fig. B*

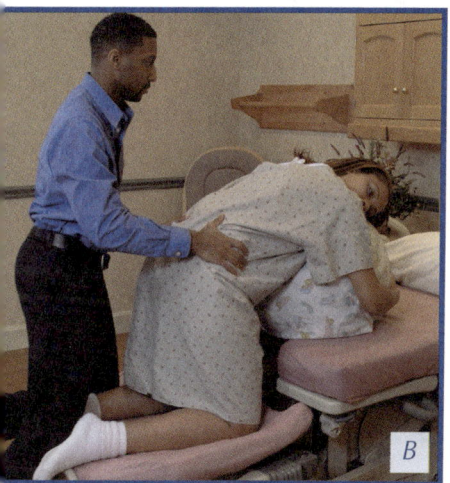

KNEE PRESSURE

Alters configuration of the pelvic basin and relieves lower back pain. Mother sits upright in a chair or lies on her side. Her partner applies pressure to her knees in the direction of her flexed hip joint. *Fig. C*

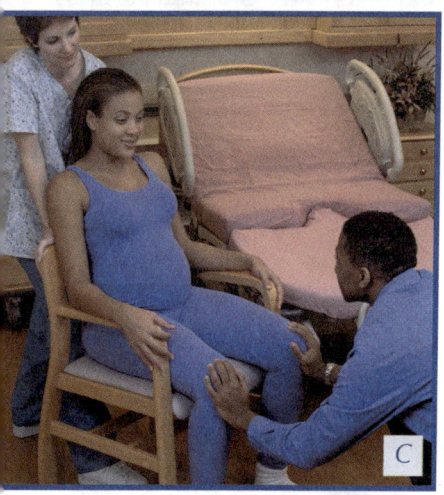

POSITIONS FOR LABOR

BACK COUNTER PRESSURE

Constant pressure applied to the sacral area of the lower back. The mother indicates where to apply the pressure and how hard. Can apply hot or cold compresses at the same time. *Fig. A*

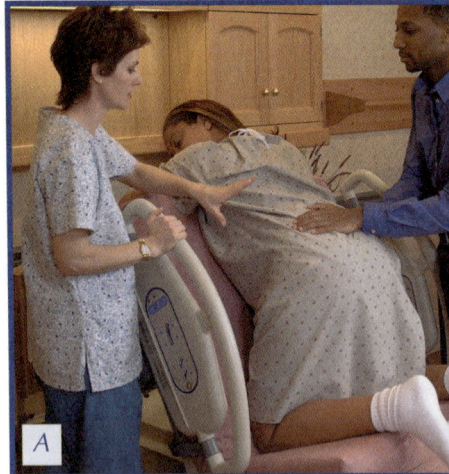

OVER HEAD OF BED

This is an alternate position for mothers who are unable to use the squatting position, or who experience back pain. The position provides easy access to a mother's lower back for massage or hot/cold compresses. *Fig. A*

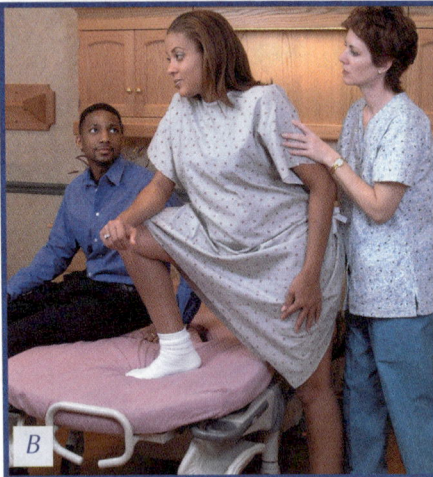

LUNGE

This position may help rotate a baby who is in an asymmetrical position. The elevated leg acts as a lever at the hip joint and enlarges the pelvis on the side where the leg is raised. *Fig. B*

EPIDURAL ANESTHESIA

The small 52 cm ball may be used in positioning patients as the epidural anesthesia is administered. *Fig. C*

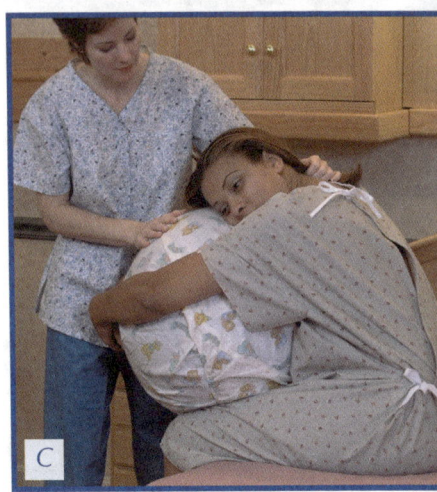

POSITIONS FOR LABOR USING A BIRTH BALL IN OR ON THE BED

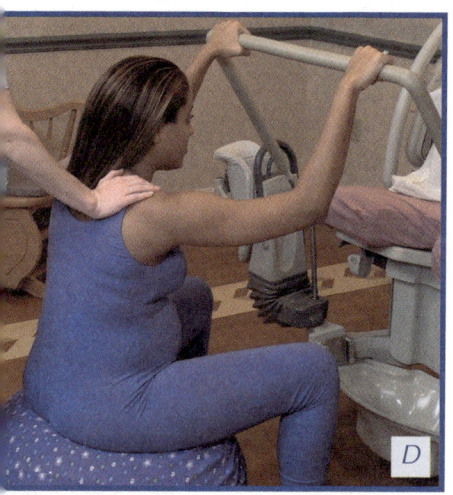

SITTING ON BALL

Elicits spontaneous movement, helps mother relax, and aids pelvic rocking. *Fig. D*

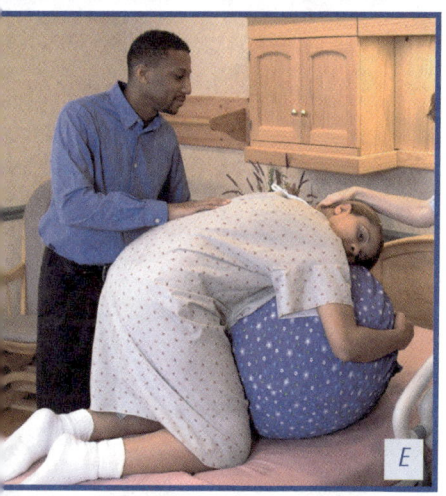

LYING ON BALL

Facilitates helpful labor positions, aids pelvic rocking and gravity. Encourages rhythmic movement. *Fig. E*

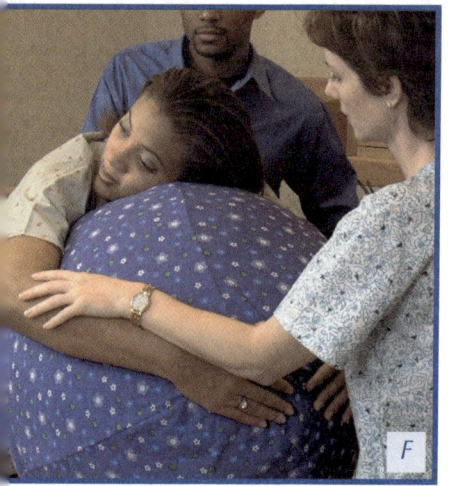

LEANING ON BALL

Leaning on the ball uses gravity to help the fetus stay in an optimal position. *Fig. F*

POSITIONS FOR LABOR

USING A PEANUT BALL DURING LABOR

Hospital labor units may choose to offer birth balls of different sizes so the caregiver can choose the best ball for an individual woman's labor. The peanut ball can be used for women who prefer a wider base of support.
Fig. A and B

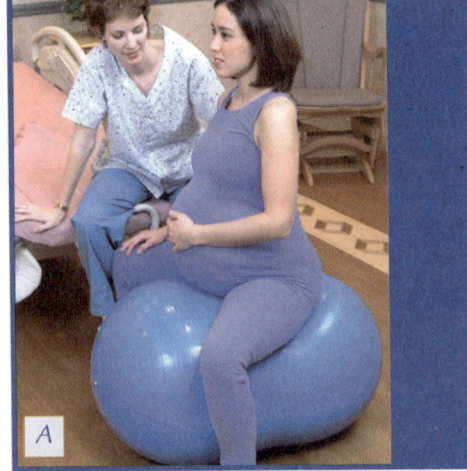

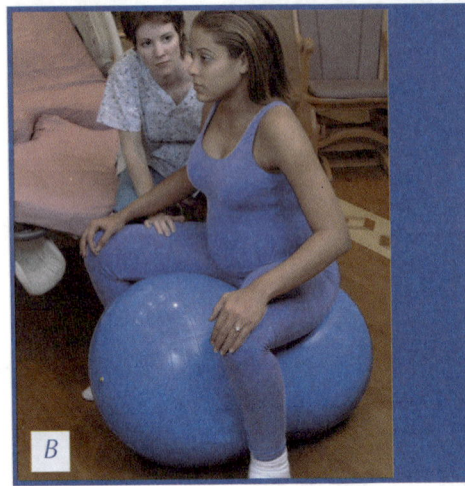

POSITIONS FOR BIRTH

SADDLE

Used if the mother experiences difficulty getting the baby under the pubic bone. The mother's feet are sole to sole and are pulled toward her as she pushes. *Fig. C*

Mothers who have epidural anesthesia should NOT use this position.

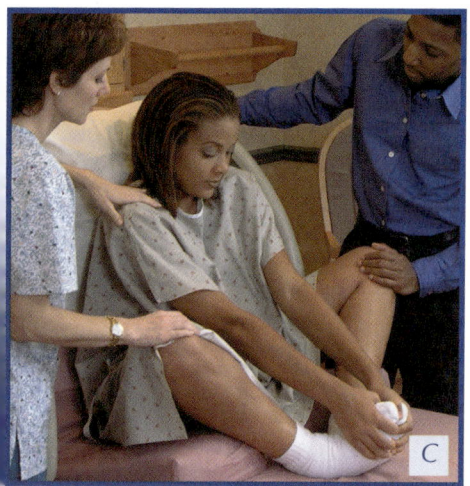

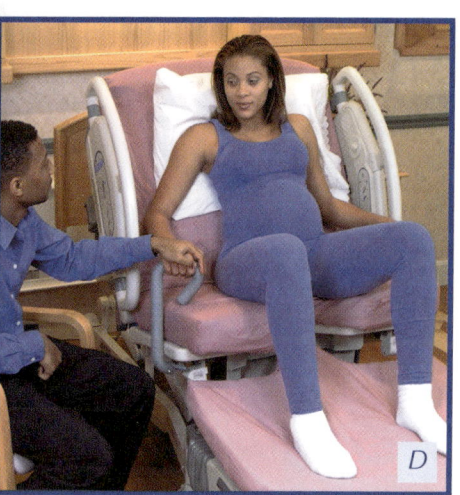

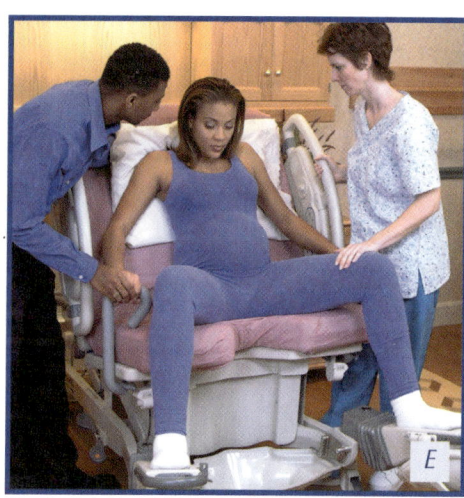

THRONE
(WITH AND WITHOUT FOOT SUPPORTS)

Mothers who have epidural anesthesia may use this position. Can provide the same benefits as the squatting position. *Fig. D and E*

33

POSITIONS FOR BIRTH USING A LABOR BAR

TUG OF WAR

May help the mother with epidural anesthesia to push more effectively by helping her control her abdominal muscles. A towel (or rubber dog chew toy) may be placed over the labor bar. The mother can pull on both ends, or the caregiver or partner can grab one end while the mother pulls. *Fig. A*

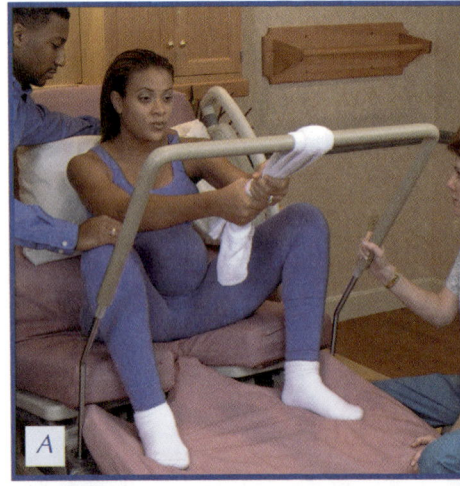

SQUATTING

May increase the diameter of the pelvis. The upper trunk pushes on the fundus, encouraging descent of the baby. May lessen mother's effort needed to push. *Fig. B*

This position may cause exhaustion and perineal floor edema. It should be used for short periods only.

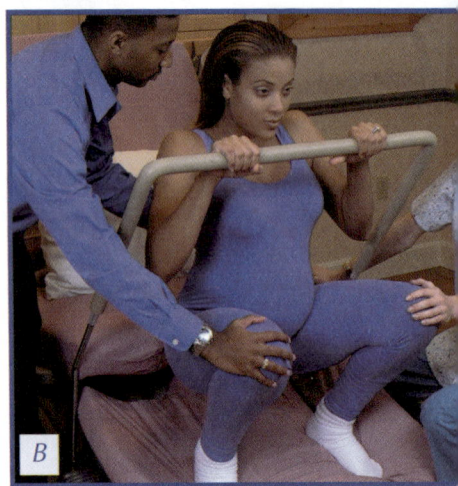

POSITIONS FOR BIRTH

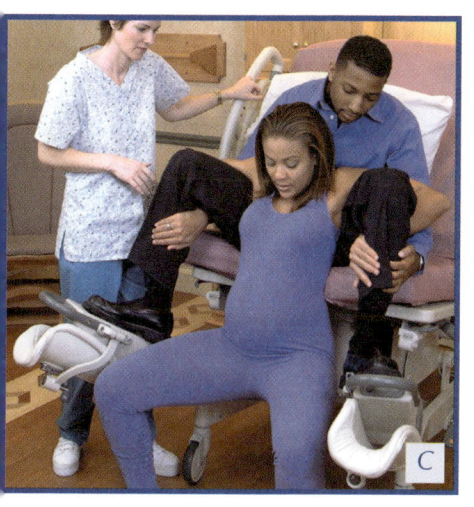

DANGLE SQUAT

Allows the partner to support all of the mother's weight. It lengthens the trunk and helps to avoid mother's unconscious tensing of abdominal muscles. *Fig. C*

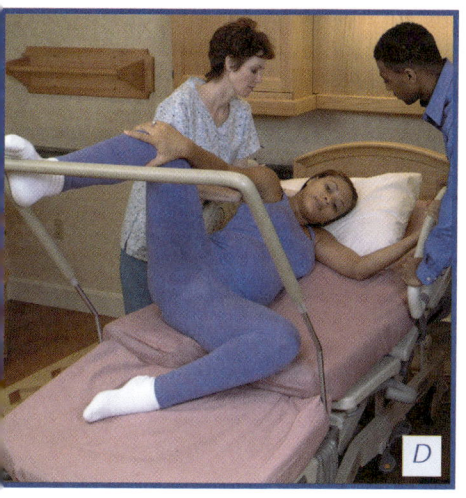

SIDE-LYING

If the mother becomes fatigued using upright positioning, she can shift to a side-lying position, either to rest between contractions or to use for support during bearing down efforts. *Fig. D*

LABOR AND THE BIRTH OF YOUR BABY

Delivering a baby is hard work! But doing some basic things to help you relax (as much as possible) and breathe well during your contractions can help decrease the discomfort you may feel. Relaxing and breathing also help provide more oxygen for you and your baby. The suggestions on the next few pages may help remind you and your support person of what you can expect during each stage of the birth journey. Use the space below to make your personal notes.

STAGES OF LABOR

THE FIRST STAGE OF LABOR—EARLY PHASE

Physical change
The first stage begins when the cervix starts to open so the baby can move into the birth canal. It ends when the cervix is 4 centimeters dilated.

What to expect
True labor contractions may start as mild cramps. They may last less than a minute and come 15 to 20 minutes apart. As time passes, the contractions come stronger and faster (3 to 5 minutes apart) and last for at least 1 minute. Your cervix begins to thin, called *efface,* and open, called *dilate*, to 4 to 5 centimeters.

What your support person can do
At Home:

- Time the contractions. Time from the beginning of one to the beginning of the next.
- Find ways for you to relax and be comfortable at home. Watch TV, listen to music, play games, or read a book to pass time. Help you get rest. You will wake up as your contractions get stronger.
- Give you clear liquids to drink.
- Help you take a warm shower so you will be more comfortable.
- Help decide when to call your care provider.
- Help when contractions are too strong to walk or talk through. Now's the time to start the breathing and relaxation techniques.
- Reassure you—your emotions will probably range from happiness that the baby is coming to fear about delivery or the baby's health. Be as positive and supportive as possible.

STAGES OF LABOR

THE FIRST STAGE OF LABOR—ACTIVE PHASE

Physical change

By now you should be in the hospital (or at least on your way). Your contractions become stronger and faster (last 1 minute and 2 to 3 minutes apart for first babies; last 1 minute and 5 minutes apart for second babies). Your cervix will thin even more and open wider, to 7 or 8 centimeters.

What to expect

You may:

- Have a backache as the baby moves lower in the birth canal
- Feel thirsty because you're breathing hard
- Feel tired

What your support person can do

- Offer words of encouragement
- Focus on labor as one contraction at a time. Each one is making the birth closer.
- Try to make you more comfortable with:
    - Cool washcloths on lips, forehead, or back of neck
    - Back or body massage
    - Warm cloths or ice packs to lower back
    - Position change
    - Lip moisturizer
- Your mood will become more serious, and you will focus more on yourself and what's happening to your body. You will also depend more on your support person.

STAGES OF LABOR

THE FIRST STAGE OF LABOR—TRANSITION PHASE

Physical change
This is the shortest phase and contractions are very strong. They are about 1 to 2 minutes apart and last about 60 seconds. This phase ends when the cervix is completely dilated.

What to expect
You may:
- Have leg cramps
- Be hot and sweaty
- Tremble
- Feel short of breath
- Feel sick to your stomach
- Feel like you have to have a bowel movement and want to push

What your support person can do
- Be as encouraging and loving as (s)he can. Remind you that soon it will be time to push and the baby will be born. Tell you, "You're almost there."
- Again, tell you to take one contraction at a time.
- For leg cramps, massage your calf, straighten the lower leg, and push toes toward your knee.
- Encourage you to puff—blow when you feel the urge to push.
- Assist you in maintaining control.

STAGES OF LABOR

THE SECOND STAGE OF LABOR

Physical change
The second stage begins when the cervix is fully dilated and effaced. It ends with the birth of your baby.

What to expect
When the cervix is completely dilated (10 centimeters), it is time to push with the contractions. Contractions are usually 2 to 5 minutes apart.

As the baby moves down, you will feel pressure on the lower back and rectum (like you are having a bowel movement). You may also feel stretching and pulling as the baby reaches the opening of your vagina and then is born.

As the birth gets closer, you will feel excited. Some women feel a renewed sense of energy and strength. Birth is an emotional experience, so don't be afraid to show your emotions (your support person too!).

To prevent your muscles from tearing and to relieve some of the pressure on your baby's head, the provider may make a small cut in the perineum (the area between your rectal and vaginal openings). (S)he will make sure the area is numb first. This is called an *episiotomy*.

THE THIRD STAGE OF LABOR

Physical change
The last stage begins after the baby is born and ends when the afterbirth, called *placenta*, is delivered.

What to expect
Shortly after the baby comes, you will feel cramping again as your placenta is delivered. After the placenta is delivered, your care provider will check you—you may need a few stitches.

Congratulations! Your labor is over. It is time now to relax and enjoy your baby. If you plan to breast feed, now is a good time to begin.

ASSISTED DELIVERY

INDUCING (STARTING) LABOR

Sometimes your care provider will want to start labor before your body starts on its own. There can be many reasons for this decision.

The night before labor is induced, you may be asked to come to the hospital. You will be given an IV and put on a monitor so your provider can watch your baby's heartbeat and your contractions. If necessary, your care provider will place medication near your cervix during a vaginal exam. You might feel some contractions after having it inserted and you might get several doses. The medication "softens" the cervix so it responds better to the Pitocin® (the medication used to induce labor).

PITOCIN® (OXYTOCIN)

If you do not need cervical softening, you will be admitted the morning of or the evening before your induction. Pitocin (oxytocin) is given through an IV to "induce" contractions. You may feel contractions after only a few minutes, or it could take several hours. Because these contractions are induced, they may be strong and uncomfortable. Don't hesitate to ask your provider for assistance.

RUPTURE OF MEMBRANE

Labor sometimes goes slowly. Your contractions may be weak or ineffective. One method used to speed up labor is to break the bag of water (rupture membranes).

VACUUM AND FORCEPS

If your pushing phase is taking too long or if the baby's condition indicates the need for a more rapid delivery, your health care provider may need to use vacuum or forcep instruments to assist you.

CESAREAN BIRTH

In cesarean birth, the baby is born through a surgical cut made through the abdomen into the uterus, or womb. There are two types of cesarean birth: planned or scheduled, and unplanned. If a cesarean birth is planned, the hospital staff will review procedures with you before your admission.

WHEN A CESAREAN IS NEEDED

Sometimes the baby is too large for the mother's pelvis, or the baby is in a position that will not allow him to be born. The mother may have a medical condition that makes immediate delivery necessary. In the midst of labor, the baby may show signs of distress or not have enough oxygen. These are examples of when a cesarean birth may be necessary.

Depending on the reason for cesarean birth, either epidural, spinal, or general anesthesia is used. With general anesthesia, your labor support partner will not be in the delivery room, since you will be asleep. If an epidural or spinal anesthetic is used, one support person may be able to stay with you.

The baby is usually born within 5 to 10 minutes after surgery begins, and the total surgery takes only about an hour. You and your support person will be given time to touch, feel, and hold the baby.

AFTER YOUR CESAREAN

During the initial recovery period, you should expect discomfort, shakes, or trembling. Most patients receive a pain medication given through the IV line which you control (PCA). Medication can also be given as a shot in your hip or arm muscle.

VAGINAL BIRTH AFTER CESAREAN (VBAC)

In the past the rule was once you had a cesarean, you always had to deliver your babies that way. Today some women who have had cesareans may try giving birth through the vagina if no risk factors are present. If you have had a previous cesarean delivery, discuss this with your care provider.

CARE AT BIRTH FOR VAGINAL, VBAC, AND C-SECTION

MOTHER'S RECOVERY CARE

After delivery your blood pressure, pulse, breathing, and temperature are checked often. In addition your episiotomy, (abdominal dressing if cesarean delivery) and vaginal bleeding are monitored.

You will be assisted by the staff when you get out of bed the first time. You will be encouraged to get up and move about within 2 hours after a vaginal delivery and within 6 to 8 hours following a cesarean section. Please ask for assistance when doing so.

Mothers are generally discharged from the hospital in a day or two. You will stay longer if you have a cesarean or complications. Rest as much as you can. The hospital staff will help you learn how to care for yourself and your baby.

REMINDERS FOR MOMS

- Call for assistance when getting up for the first time after delivery.
- Keep your call light within easy reach. Don't push yourself to the point of fatigue.
- Request pain medication when needed.
- Use your call light if you or your baby need help.
- If you feel drowsy or sleepy when holding your baby, place your baby in a bassinet or crib. Falling asleep in a chair or in bed while holding a baby can be dangerous. Babies may fall, suffocate, or become injured.
- Wear a supportive bra after delivery. It will help keep your breasts from becoming too uncomfortable.

BABY'S MEDICAL CARE AT BIRTH

In the birthing or delivery room, your baby's umbilical cord is clamped. The baby is dried and wrapped in a blanket. Your baby will be given a bath when he is warm and stable.

- All newborns are slightly low on vitamin K, which is necessary for normal blood clotting. Your baby will be given an injection of this vitamin to prevent bleeding.

- Eye infections that can be contracted as your baby passes through the birth canal are also a danger. Erythromycin eye ointment is placed on your baby's eyes to prevent infection.

- Your newborn may also be given his first hepatitis B vaccination, with your consent. This series of three immunizations is given during baby's first six months to prevent a virus that causes serious liver disease.

- Some states require a hearing screening for all newborns.

A provider who specializes in baby care will examine your baby more thoroughly during your hospital stay. You can choose this doctor in advance and list the name on the admission form. Otherwise the hospital will assign one. Your baby should see the doctor again when he is about 2 weeks old, unless you are told to come sooner.

WHILE IN THE HOSPITAL

IDENTIFICATION AND INFANT SECURITY

The safety and protection of your baby are of utmost importance to our staff. Various measures have been put into place to help prevent unauthorized access to your baby. Our staff will explain this system to you when you arrive on the unit.

BIRTH CERTIFICATE AND SOCIAL SECURITY NUMBER

During your hospital stay, a staff member will ask you to fill out information for your baby's birth certificate. Please have the following information ready:

- Correct spelling of baby's name

- Mother's maiden name (the name you had before you were married), date and place of birth, Social Security number

- Father's full name, date and place of birth, and Social Security number

- For unmarried couples, an affidavit of parentage must be completed for the name of the baby's father to be included on the birth certificate.

Young children need Social Security numbers for many reasons. If you plan to open a bank account, buy savings bonds, or apply for some kinds of government services for your child, your child will need a number. And since 1988 any children who are age 2 or older must have Social Security numbers in order for you to claim them as dependents on your Federal income tax return. The Internal Revenue Service (IRS) may use Social Security information to verify your earned income tax credits.

Call the state department of vital records if you have questions about the birth certificate. Call 1-800-772-1213 if you have questions about the Social Security number.

MOM'S CARE AT HOME

Your body and emotions are both adjusting to the birth, which is, after all, a tremendous event. Be patient with yourself, your partner, and your baby.

Most new mothers feel upset at times—angry, sad, or overwhelmed. This is common; not only is a new baby a huge responsibility, but a new mother often feels physically drained from the effort of carrying and then delivering a child. Plus, your hormones are adjusting, which can cause mood swings. Not getting enough sleep adds to these feelings.

Such feelings are troubling, but may be normal. They usually go away within a few hours or at most, in one or two weeks.

Here are some steps that may help you take care of yourself during these hectic days.

- Nurture yourself physically. Get rest. Exercise regularly.
- Develop a support system—family, friends, other mothers.
- Express and accept your feelings, both positive and negative.
- Take breaks. Do something you enjoy.
- Keep your expectations realistic.
- Enjoy or laugh at something each day.
- Plan your day.
- Postpone major life changes.

The blues are one thing. Full-fledged depression is another. If you think you need help, do not hesitate—call your health care provider right away. Help is available to get you through a difficult time.

DEPRESSION

A prolonged period of "the blues" or more severe depression may occur and is cause for concern. If a woman is so depressed she can't function normally, she needs help. If you have some of the problems listed below, talk to your care provider at once.

- Depression or "the blues" that lasts more than two weeks
- Severe anger and sadness that comes on a month or two after the baby is born
- Feelings of sadness, doubt, guilt, or helplessness that seem to increase each week
- Difficulty concentrating or remembering. Trouble doing tasks at home or on the job. Not able to care for yourself or your baby.
- Anxiety or panic attacks
- Extreme behavior:
    - Unable to sleep even when tired, or a wish to sleep all the time
    - Wanting to eat all day long, or never wanting to eat
    - Extreme worry about the baby, or no interest at all in the baby or the rest of the family or activities that you normally enjoy
    - Having thoughts about harming yourself or your baby

POSTPARTUM DEPRESSION RESOURCES

These publications can provide more information about postpartum depression:

Postpartum Depression: Every Woman's Guide to Diagnosis, Treatment and Prevention, by Sharon I. Roan

Depression After Childbirth, by Katharina Dalton

Mothering the New Mother, by Sally Placksin

The Year After Childbirth, by Sheila Kitzinger

This organization can help you find a support group:

Postpartum Support International
927 N. Kellogg, Santa Barbara, CA 93111
Telephone: 1-805-967-7636
Fax: 1-805-967-0608
Internet: www.iup.edu/an/postpartum/

WARNING SIGNS TO WATCH FOR

There are some things you may notice that are NOT normal. They could be your body's way of saying there is a problem. Call your care provider if you notice any of these warning signs.

- fever of 100.4°F or higher
- nausea and vomiting
- pain or burning when you empty your bladder, frequent urination, or urgency (sudden, strong desire to urinate)
- heavy, bright-red bleeding or large clots
- pain, swelling, or tenderness in the legs
- chest pain and cough
- hot, tender, reddened areas or painful lumps in the breast
- painful cramps or abdominal pain
- increased pain in your episiotomy (stitches)
- C-section incision that is red, hot, more painful, drains fluid, or opens up
- feelings that you might harm yourself or your baby
- feeling so sad or depressed you cannot take care of yourself or baby
- severe headache that medicine does not relieve
- flu symptoms (fever, body aches, headache, or nausea)
- constipation that diet or stool softeners do not relieve

NUTRITION

HEALTHY EATING

Eat a variety of healthy foods and drink 6 to 8 glasses of water or liquids a day, just as when you were pregnant.

If you have questions about what you should eat, ask your care provider.

If you are breastfeeding, good nutrition is important for you and your baby. Stay away from caffeine, alcohol, tobacco, and drugs. You will need an extra 500 calories a day from the basic food groups. Continue taking your prenatal vitamins.

FOOD PYRAMID

All new mothers and their families need a healthy diet of a variety of foods. Mothers who breastfeed need to eat healthy so they have a good supply of high-quality milk. The Food Pyramid on Appendix A, page 58, shows the recommended amount of each food group for you and your family.

ACTIVITY LEVEL AND EXERCISE

Your activity level should be based on the idea that physical activity is not harmful. As a rule, gradually increase your activity from day to day and do more things as you feel like it. Here are some basic guidelines:

- Gradually resume activities
- No heavy lifting—nothing over 20 pounds, especially if you had a cesarean delivery
- No driving for two weeks after a cesarean delivery. This is especially important if you are feeling weak or taking pain medication. Get clearance from your care provider before you begin driving.

POSTPARTUM FITNESS EXERCISES AFTER DELIVERY SUGGESTED BY ACOG

Exercise will help you get back in shape. You should consult your doctor about any exercises, especially if you had a cesarean delivery.

The 6 fitness exercises that follow are suggested by the American College of Obstetricians and Gynecologists for new mothers. However, you should always consult your health care provider before you begin any personal fitness or exercise program.

American College of Obstetricians and Gynecologists: Planning for Pregnancy, Birth and Beyond, Second Edition © 1995 and Third Edition © 2000. Washington, DC, ACOG. Used with permission.

LEG SLIDES

This simple exercise tones abdominal and leg muscles. It does not put much strain on your incision if you have had a cesarean birth. You should try to repeat this exercise several times a day.

- Lie flat on your back and bend your knees slightly.
- Inhale, slide your right leg from a bent to a straight position, exhale, and bend it back again.
- Be sure that you keep both feet on the floor and keep them relaxed.
- Repeat with your left leg.

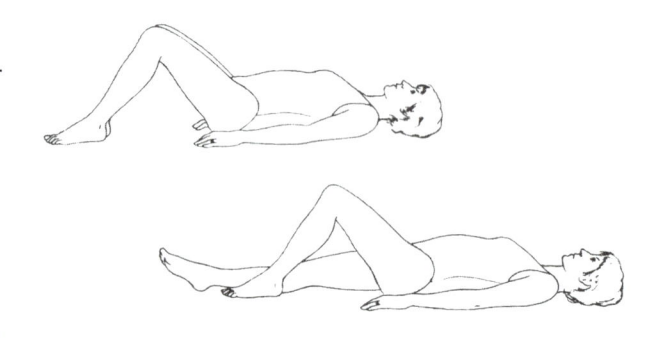

HEAD LIFTS

Head lifts can progress to shoulder lifts and curl-ups, all of which strengthen the abdominal muscles. When you feel comfortable doing 10 head lifts at a time, proceed to shoulder lifts. (If you had a cesarean birth, ask your health care provider before progressing beyond head lifts.)

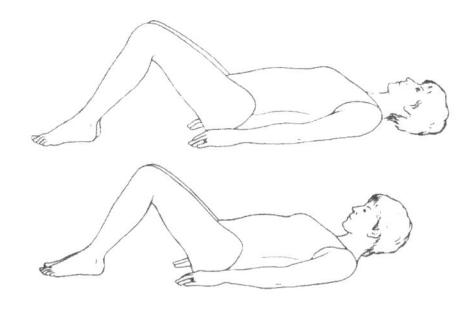

- Lie on your back with your arms along your sides. Bend your knees so that your feet are flat on the floor.
- Inhale and relax your abdomen.
- Exhale slowly as you lift your head off the floor.
- Inhale as you lower your head again.

SHOULDER LIFTS

Begin the same way as you would for head lifts. When you feel comfortable doing 10 shoulder lifts at a time, proceed with curl-ups.

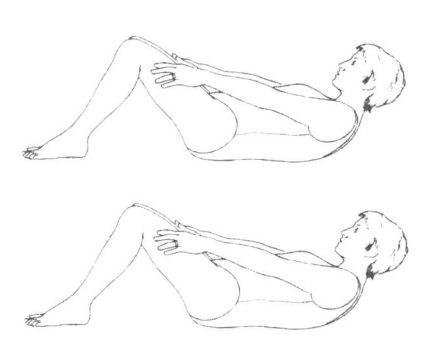

- Inhale and relax your abdomen.
- Exhale slowly and lift your head and shoulders off the floor. Reach with your arms so that you don't use them for support.
- Inhale as you lower your shoulders to the floor.

POSTPARTUM FITNESS EXERCISES SUGGESTED BY ACOG

CURL-UPS

Begin the same way as you would for head lifts, lying on your back with your knees bent and your arms at your sides. Keep your lower back flat on the floor.

- Inhale, relaxing your abdomen.
- Exhale. Reach with your arms, and slowly raise your torso to the point halfway between your knees and the floor (about a 45° angle).
- Inhale as you lower yourself to the floor.

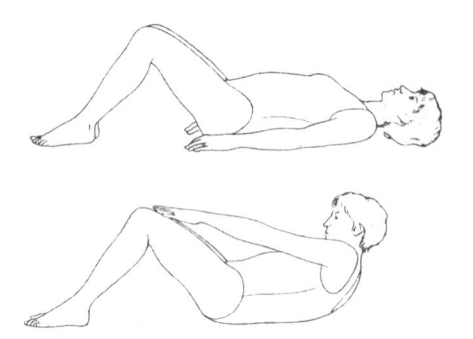

KNEELING PELVIC TILT

Tilting your pelvis back toward your spine helps strengthen your abdominal muscles.

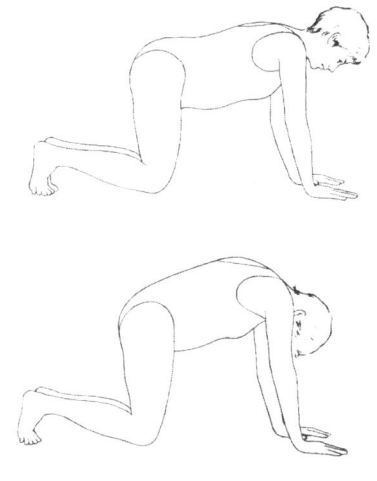

- Begin on your hands and knees. Your back should be relaxed, not curved or arched.
- Inhale.
- Exhale and pull your buttocks forward, rotating the pubic bone upward.
- Hold for a count of 3, then inhale and relax.
- Repeat 5 times and add 1 or 2 repetitions a day if you can.

KEGEL EXERCISES

Kegel exercises tone your pelvic-floor muscles. This, in turn, controls bladder leaks, helps the perineum heal, and tightens a vagina stretched from birth.

- Squeeze the muscles that you use to stop the flow of urine.
- Hold for up to 10 seconds, then release.
- Do this 10-20 times in a row at least three times a day.

BIRTH BALL EXERCISES POSTPARTUM

Some childbirth specialists recommend the use of the ball postpartum (after delivery).

PELVIC LIFT EXERCISE

Lying flat with the ball under the calves, lift hips off the floor and hold. Then release, lowering the hips and return to the starting position.
Fig. A and B

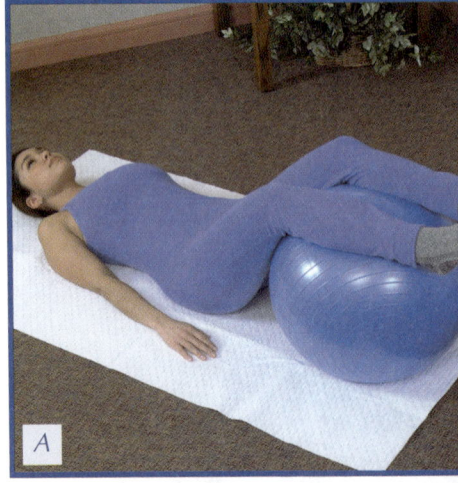

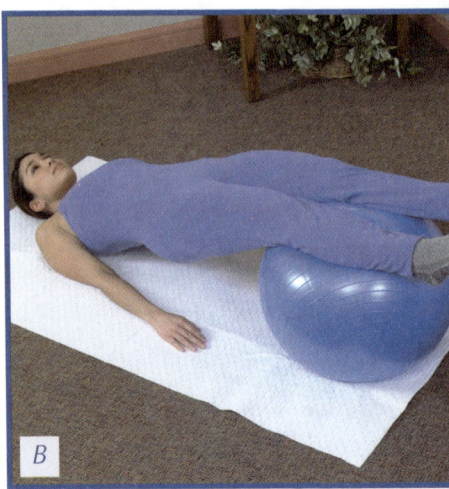

LUNGE

Push the ball against a flat wall with your back. Slowly lower to a sitting position, rolling the ball down the wall with your back. Stop when your thighs are parallel to the floor or higher. Your knees should be directly over your feet, your heels planted firmly on the floor. Return to an upright position and repeat.
Fig. C and D

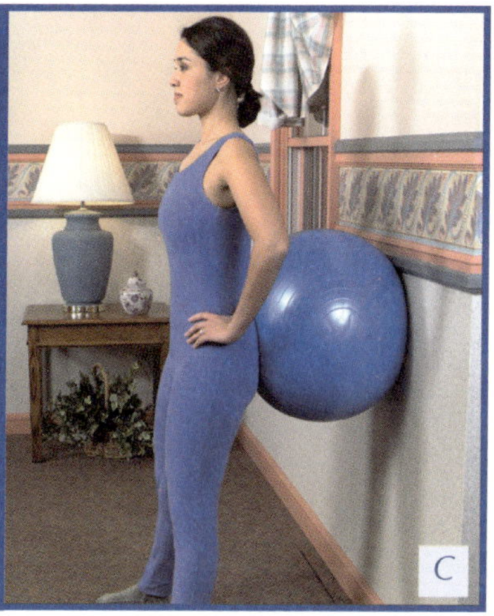

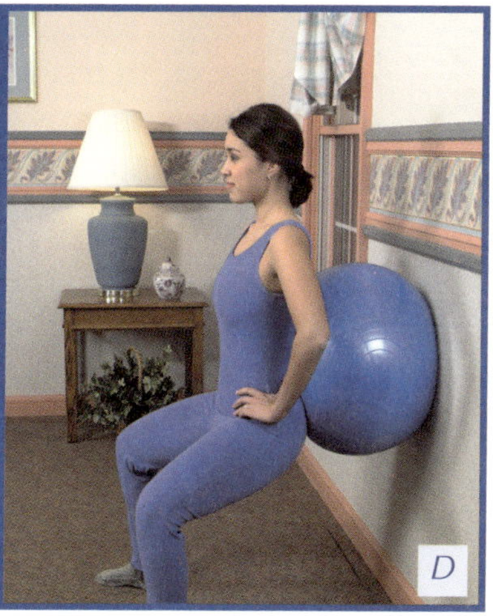

PERSONAL NOTES

APPENDICES

APPENDIX A: FOOD PYRAMID

All new mothers and their families need a healthy diet of a variety of foods. Mothers who breastfeed need to eat healthy so they have a good supply of high-quality milk. The number of servings printed in bold under each group name are for your family.

SOURCE: U.S. Department of Agriculture and U.S. Department of Health and Human Services

Milk, Yogurt & Cheese Group
2 - 3 servings
Pregnant Women: 3 - 4 servings
Breastfeeding Women: 3 - 4 servings
Postpartum Women: 2 - 3 servings
Pregnant/Breastfeeding Teens: 4 servings

What Counts as A Serving?
1 cup milk or yogurt; 1½ oz. natural or 2 oz. processed cheese; ½ cup ice cream, ice milk, or frozen yogurt

Vegetable Group
3 - 5 servings

What Counts as A Serving?
1 cup raw leafy greens; ½ cup cooked or chopped raw veggies; ½ cup vegetable juice; 1 medium tomato; 1 medium potato; 5 asparagus spears; 7 carrot sticks; 1 ear of corn on the cob

Bread, Cereal, Rice & Pasta Group
6 - 11 servings
Pregnant women: 8 - 11 servings

What Counts as a Serving? Don't confuse a serving with a helping of food. For example, the servings in a dressed cheeseburger include:

- 2 servings of bread • 1 serving of meat • ½ serving of cheese
- ½ serving of vegetable (lettuce, tomato, onion)

Fats, Oils & Sweets
Use sparingly

Meat, Poultry, Fish, Dry Beans, Eggs & Nuts Group
2 - 3 servings
Pregnant Women: 3 servings
Breastfeeding Women: 2 - 3 servings
Postpartum Women: 2 - 3 servings

What Counts as A Serving?
2-3 oz. cooked lean meat, poultry, or fish,
OR foods that count as 1 oz. of meat like
½ cup cooked dry beans; 1 egg; ⅓ cup nuts;
2 tablespoons peanut butter

Fruit Group
2 - 4 servings

What Counts as A Serving?
1 medium apple, banana, orange, peach;
2 medium plums or tangerines;
⅓ cantaloupe; 15 small grapes;
½ cup cut-up raw or canned fruit;
½ cup fruit juice; 8 medium strawberries; ½ cup blueberries;
½ avocado

What Counts as A Serving?
1 slice bread; 1 English muffin; ½ bagel;
1 oz. dry cereal; ½ cup cooked cereal, rice, or
pasta; 5-6 small crackers; 2 cookies

APPENDIX B: GLOSSARY

Here are some medical terms your care givers may use.

AMNIOTIC FLUID: Fluid found in the membrane sac, or bag of waters, which surrounds the baby in the uterus. It acts as a cushion and warms the baby during pregnancy.

AMNIOTOMY: Artificial rupturing of the amniotic sac surrounding baby.

AUGMENTATION OF LABOR: Increasing the strength of labor contractions after labor has begun by giving Pitocin through an IV.

BACK LABOR: Labor felt in the lower back, buttocks, and thighs. Often caused by the position of the baby or the anatomy of the mother. Can be painful. Try position changes, counterpressure, or massage for relief.

BIRTH CANAL: The passageway from the cervix through the vagina.

BRAXTON-HICKS CONTRACTIONS: Intermittent uterine contractions present throughout pregnancy. They can become stronger or more frequent in the last months as the uterus is preparing itself for labor. The cervix does not efface (thin) or dilate (open) with these contractions.

BREECH: Delivery of the baby with the buttocks or feet first.

CERVIX: Lower end of the uterus. It effaces (thins) and dilates (opens) in response to labor contractions.

CESAREAN BIRTH: Surgical delivery of the baby through the abdominal and uterine walls.

CONTRACTIONS: The rhythmical tightening and relaxation of the uterine muscles. During "true" labor, contractions cause the cervix to efface and dilate and help push the baby down and out.

CROWNING: When the presenting part of the baby (usually the crown of the head) is visible at the vaginal opening just before birth.

DILATION: The gradual opening of the cervix to allow the baby to move into the vagina. It is measured from 0 to 10 centimeters.

EFFACEMENT: Gradual thinning and shortening of the cervix. Effacement is measured in percentages, from 0% to 100%.

EFFLEURAGE: Light massage over the abdomen during labor for relaxation.

ENGAGEMENT: When the presenting part of the baby has descended into the opening of the mother's pelvic bone.

EPISIOTOMY: A surgical incision made into the perineum before delivery that enlarges the vaginal opening for delivery of the baby.

FETAL MONITOR: A machine used to detect and record uterine contractions and the baby's heart rate.

FORCEPS: Two tong-shaped metal guides which are placed inside the birth canal, one along each side of the baby's head. Forceps help the baby through the birth canal when the mother has difficulty pushing baby out.

FUNDUS: The upper, rounded portion of the uterus.

INDUCTION: The use of medications and/or rupture of membranes to start uterine contractions.

IV: Intravenous infusion. Needle and tubing inserted into a vein in order to give medication or fluids.

LABOR: Rhythmical series of contractions which increase in strength, frequency, and duration and cause the cervix to dilate and efface.

LIGHTENING: The sensation of the baby "dropping" as the baby descends into the pelvic cavity.

MEMBRANE: Membranous sac or bag which contains amniotic fluid. Also known as amniotic sac or bag of waters.

MUCOUS PLUG: A thick plug which blocks the cervical canal during pregnancy. It protects the uterus from bacteria present in the vagina. Sometimes called *bloody show* because it may have streaks of blood mixed with the mucous.

PELVIS: The basin-shaped ring of bones made up of the hip bones, pubic bones, and sacrum. The baby passes through this ring during birth.

PERINEUM: Skin and muscle surrounding the vagina and rectum.

PLACENTA: The organ attached to the wall of the uterus and connected to the baby by the umbilical cord. The placenta gives the baby nutrition and processes her wastes. Pushed out after labor, it is called *afterbirth*.

POSTPARTUM: After delivery. The period between childbirth and return of the uterus to normal size—approximately six weeks.

UMBILICAL CORD: Composed of two arteries and one vein, this cord connects the baby to the placenta. Surrounded by a jelly-like material called *Wharton's Jelly*.

UTERUS: The muscular reproductive organ in which the baby grows and develops during pregnancy. It contracts during labor to move the baby through the birth canal for delivery. Also called *womb*.

VACUUM EXTRACTION: Gentle suction through a soft rubber cap on the baby's head which helps the doctor deliver the baby when the mother is having difficulty pushing the baby out. Used instead of forceps.

VBAC: Vaginal Birth After Cesarean section.

INDEX

A
Afterbirth..................................40
Anatomy of pregnancy 6
Aromatherapy 28
Assisted delivery..........................41

B
Baby's medical care at birth 44
Bag of waters 24, 26
Birth ball
    During pregnancy 14-17
    During labor and delivery....29-32
    After delivery 55
Birth certificate 45
Birth comfort positions
    Dangle squat.............................35
    Saddle.......................................33
    Side-lying.................................35
    Squatting 34
    Throne 33
    Tug of war 34
Bloody show 24
Bowel movement change 24
Braxton-Hicks contractions 25

C
Care at birth 43
Cesarean birth 42
Checklist before delivery 18
Comfort measures 28
    Aromatherapy...........................28
    Hydrotherapy 28
    Sterile water injections..............28
    See "Birth comfort positions"
    and "Labor comfort positions"
Coming to the hospital 27
    Admission 27
    Care team 27
Contractions 24-25, 37-40

D
Decisions before you deliver 18
Depression....................................47
Dilation 37

E
Eating out 7
Effacement 24, 37
Episiotomy 40, 43
Erythromycin 44
Exercise
    Importance of............................9
    Warning signs...........................9
    ACOG exercises
        Pregnancy.......................10-13
        Postpartum 50-53
Labor ball
    First trimester 14
    Second trimester 15
    Third trimester.....................17

F
False labor....................................25
Food pyramid 58
Forceps 41

G
Glossary 60

H
Healthy eating
    Pregnancy..................................7
    After you deliver 49
Hepatitis B vaccine 44
Hospital
    Admission 27
    Identification 45
    Infant security 45
Hydrotherapy 28

I
Inducing (starting) labor 41

K
Kegel exercises 53

L
Labor
    Signs of labor 24
    True vs false labor 25
    When labor starts 26
    Also see "Stages of labor"
Labor comfort positions
    Back counter pressure 30
    Double hip squeeze 29
    Epidural anesthesia 30
    Knee pressure 29
    Leaning on ball 31
    Lunge 30
    Lying on ball 31
    Over head of bed 30
    Sitting on ball 31
Lightening 24
Low backaches 24

M
Mother's care at home
    Tips for first days 46
    Depression 47
    Warning signs 48
Mother's hospital recovery care 43

N
Nesting 24
Nutrition
    During pregnancy 7
    After delivery (postpartum) 49

O
Oxytocin 41

P
Packing for the hospital 21
Pitocin 41
Placenta 40
Planning for hospital visitors 19
Postpartum depression 47

R
Rupture of membrane 41

S
Security for infant in hospital 45
Shopping lists 20
Signs of labor 24
Social Security number 45
Stages of labor
    First stage 37-39
        Early phase 37
        Active phase 38
        Transition phase 39
    Second stage 40
    Third stage 40
Sterile water injections 28

T
To-do checklist 18

V
Vacuum cup 41
Vaginal Birth After Delivery 43
Vitamin K 44

W
Warning signs
    After delivery 48
Weight gain 8
What to bring to the hospital 21